PDA Autism and the Family

The Handbook for Understanding, Supporting, and Embracing Your Unique Family Dynamics with Humor and Compassion

Liz Adet

Copyright © 2024 by Liz Adet

All rights reserved. No part of this book may be reproduced, stored in a retrieval system, or transmitted in any form or by any means, electronic, mechanical, photocopying, recording, or otherwise, without prior written permission from the author, except for brief quotations in critical reviews or articles

Table of Contents

Introduction	1
Chapter 1	3
Understanding PDA Autism	3
What is PDA Autism?	3
Characteristics and Traits	4
Diagnosis and Assessment	6
Impact on Family Dynamics	8
Chapter 2	11
Exploring Family Dynamics	11
Family Systems Theory	11
Roles Within the Family	13
Communication Challenges	15
Coping Mechanisms	18
Chapter 3	21
Navigating Daily Life	21
Routines and Flexibility	21
Sensory Sensitivities	22
Emotional Regulation	24
School and Education	26
Chapter 4	29
Supporting Your Child	29
Parenting Strategies	29
Building Self-Esteem	31
Advocating for Your Child	33
Accessing Resources and Support Services	35
Chapter 5	39
Sibling Relationships	39

Understanding Sibling Dynamics	39
Supporting Siblings	40
Building Strong Bonds	42
Addressing Sibling Challenges	44
Chapter 6	**47**
Partner Support	**47**
Maintaining Connection	47
Coping Strategies for Couples	49
Balancing Responsibilities	51
Seeking External Support	52
Chapter 7	**55**
Extended Family and Community	**55**
Educating Extended Family Members	55
Creating Supportive Networks	58
Community Resources and Programs	60
Advocating for Awareness and Understanding	63
Chapter 8	**66**
Embracing Humor and Compassion	**66**
Finding Joy in Everyday Moments	66
Celebrating Differences	67
Fostering Resilience	69
Cultivating a Positive Outlook	71
Conclusion	**74**

Introduction

Within the realm of neurodevelopmental disorders, Pathological Demand Avoidance (PDA) Autism stands as a distinct yet complex condition, presenting unique challenges and dynamics within family units. This handbook, **"PDA Autism and the Family**," serves as a comprehensive guide crafted to offer understanding, support, and compassion to families navigating the complexities of PDA Autism.

Welcome to a journey of understanding, supporting, and embracing the unique dynamics of PDA Autism within the family. Imagine embarking on an adventure where every twist and turn offers a new opportunity for growth, connection, and discovery. In this handbook, we'll navigate through the world of PDA Autism with curiosity, empathy, and a touch of humor.

Picture a family setting out on a quest, armed not with swords and shields, but with love, compassion, and resilience. Each member of the family brings their own strengths and challenges to the journey, creating a mosaic of experiences, emotions, and perspectives. Together, they navigate the uncharted territories of PDA Autism, seeking understanding, support, and acceptance along the way.

As you embark on this journey together, you'll explore the diverse nature of PDA Autism, from its unique characteristics and impact on family dynamics to practical strategies for navigating daily life and fostering support networks. Through engaging anecdotes, relatable scenarios, and practical advice, we'll uncover the joys, challenges, and triumphs of life with PDA Autism.

Get ready to embark on an adventure filled with laughter, tears, and moments of profound insight. You'll navigate the twists and turns of the PDA Autism journey with courage, compassion, and a sense of wonder. So grab your map, pack your bags, and get ready for an unforgettable journey into the world of PDA Autism. The adventure awaits!

Chapter 1

Understanding PDA Autism

What is PDA Autism?

Pathological Demand Avoidance (PDA) Autism, also known as Extreme Demand Avoidance (EDA) Autism, is a subtype of autism spectrum disorder (ASD) characterized by a profound difficulty with managing and responding to demands and expectations placed upon an individual. Unlike traditional autism, individuals with PDA Autism exhibit a pervasive need to resist and avoid everyday demands and requests, often displaying high levels of anxiety and a strong desire for control. PDA Autism was first identified and described by Elizabeth Newson in the 1980s and has since garnered recognition as a distinct profile within the autism spectrum.

Central to the concept of PDA Autism is the notion of demand avoidance, which manifests in a variety of contexts, including social interactions, academic settings, and daily routines. Individuals with PDA Autism often employ complex and elaborate strategies to resist demands, such as negotiation, distraction, or defiance, in an attempt to regain a sense of control over their environment. This pervasive avoidance of demands can significantly impact various aspects of an individual's life, including their ability to form relationships, participate in educational or vocational activities, and engage in daily routines.

It's important to note that while individuals with PDA Autism share commonalities with those diagnosed with traditional autism, there are distinct differences in their presentation and responses to intervention. Understanding these differences is crucial for providing tailored support and accommodations that address the unique needs of individuals with PDA Autism and their families.

Characteristics and Traits

The characteristics and traits associated with PDA Autism encompass a broad spectrum of behaviors and challenges that profoundly impact an individual's functioning and well-being. At the core of PDA Autism is a pervasive difficulty with managing and responding to demands, which often leads to a range of adaptive and maladaptive coping strategies.

One of the hallmark characteristics of PDA Autism is the use of social manipulation and avoidance techniques to evade demands and maintain a sense of control. Individuals may employ strategies such as appearing compliant while covertly resisting or avoiding tasks, or engaging in elaborate negotiation tactics to deflect requests. This complex interplay between compliance and resistance can often confound caregivers and educators, making it challenging to discern genuine capabilities and needs.

In addition to demand avoidance, individuals with PDA Autism may exhibit heightened levels of anxiety and emotional dysregulation in response to perceived demands or expectations. This emotional intensity can manifest in meltdowns, tantrums, or withdrawal behaviors, further complicating social interactions and daily functioning. Furthermore, individuals with PDA Autism may display an exceptional level of social cognition and empathy, despite their difficulties with social interaction, leading to a paradoxical combination of social adeptness and avoidance.

Other common characteristics of PDA Autism include a preference for routine and sameness, sensory sensitivities, and a strong need for autonomy and control over their environment. These traits, when viewed in conjunction with demand avoidance and emotional dysregulation, contribute to the complex and multifaceted nature of PDA Autism.

Diagnosis and Assessment

The diagnosis and assessment of PDA Autism pose significant challenges due to the unique and nuanced nature of the condition. Unlike traditional autism, which is characterized by a more standardized set of diagnostic criteria, PDA Autism lacks clear-cut guidelines for identification and classification. As a result, clinicians and diagnosticians often rely on a combination of behavioral observations, developmental history, and standardized assessments to make an accurate diagnosis.

One of the primary challenges in diagnosing PDA Autism lies in differentiating it from other conditions with overlapping features, such as oppositional defiant disorder (ODD), attention-deficit/hyperactivity disorder (ADHD), or anxiety disorders. Individuals with PDA Autism may exhibit behaviors commonly associated with these conditions, further complicating the diagnostic process.

To aid in the assessment of PDA Autism, clinicians may utilize specialized tools and measures designed to capture the unique features of the condition. These assessments may include structured interviews with caregivers and teachers, behavioral observations in various settings, and standardized measures of social communication and adaptive functioning. Additionally, a thorough evaluation of co-occurring conditions, such as sensory processing difficulties or anxiety, is essential for comprehensive diagnosis and intervention planning.

It's important to approach the diagnostic process with sensitivity and flexibility, recognizing that individuals with PDA Autism may present with a diverse range of strengths and challenges that defy easy categorization. A multidisciplinary approach, involving collaboration between clinicians, educators, and caregivers, can facilitate a more comprehensive understanding of an individual's needs and inform targeted interventions and support strategies.

Impact on Family Dynamics

The impact of PDA Autism on family dynamics is profound and multifaceted, influencing the emotional, social, and practical aspects of daily life for all members of the family unit. From the moment of diagnosis, families are thrust into a journey marked by uncertainty, advocacy, and adaptation as they navigate the unique challenges posed by PDA Autism.

One of the primary challenges faced by families living with PDA Autism is the pervasive nature of demand avoidance and its ripple effects on daily routines and interactions. The constant negotiation and management of demands can create a highly volatile and unpredictable environment, leading to heightened stress and anxiety for both individuals with PDA Autism and their caregivers. As a result, family members may find themselves constantly on edge, anticipating and navigating potential triggers and meltdowns.

Furthermore, the emotional intensity and dysregulation commonly associated with PDA Autism can strain familial relationships and communication dynamics. Caregivers may struggle to understand and respond effectively to the emotional needs of their loved ones, while siblings may feel overlooked or overwhelmed by the demands placed on the family unit. This dynamic can lead to feelings of isolation, guilt, and frustration among family members, further exacerbating the challenges of living with PDA Autism.

In addition to the emotional impact, PDA Autism can also have practical implications for family functioning, including difficulties with accessing appropriate services and supports, managing transitions and changes in routine, and balancing caregiving responsibilities with other commitments. Navigating these practical challenges requires resilience, creativity, and a strong support network to ensure the well-being of both individuals with PDA Autism and their families.

Despite the profound challenges posed by PDA Autism, many families find strength and resilience in their shared journey, drawing upon humor, compassion, and mutual support to navigate the ups and downs of daily life. By fostering open communication, empathy, and a willingness to adapt and learn, families can create a nurturing and inclusive environment where individuals with PDA Autism can thrive and fulfill their potential.

Chapter 2

Exploring Family Dynamics

Family Systems Theory

Family Systems Theory, developed by Murray Bowen in the 1950s, offers a comprehensive framework for understanding the complex interactions and dynamics within family units. At its core, Family Systems Theory posits that families operate as interconnected and interdependent systems, wherein each member plays a role in shaping and maintaining the overall functioning of the family unit. Central to this theory is the concept of differentiation, which refers to the degree to which individuals can maintain their sense of self while remaining emotionally connected to the family system.

In the context of PDA Autism, Family Systems Theory provides valuable insights into the ways in which family dynamics may be influenced and shaped by the presence of a member with PDA Autism. The demands and challenges associated with PDA Autism can disrupt the equilibrium of the family system, leading to shifts in roles, communication patterns, and relational dynamics. Understanding these dynamics through the lens of Family Systems Theory can empower families to identify areas of strength and resilience, as well as areas in need of support and intervention.

One of the key principles of Family Systems Theory is the notion of triangulation, wherein conflicts or tensions between two individuals are often mediated or diffused through the involvement of a third party. In families affected by PDA Autism, triangulation may manifest in various ways, such as the triangulation of parental conflicts through the child with PDA Autism, or the triangulation of sibling relationships around the needs and demands of the individual with PDA Autism. Recognizing and addressing these patterns of triangulation is essential for promoting healthy communication and problem-solving within the family system.

Furthermore, Family Systems Theory emphasizes the importance of boundaries within family units, both in terms of physical space and emotional autonomy. Individuals with PDA Autism may struggle with boundary regulation, either by enacting rigid and inflexible boundaries or by intruding upon the boundaries of others. This dynamic can create tension and conflict within the family system, as members navigate the delicate balance between autonomy and connectedness. By fostering clear and flexible boundaries, families can create a supportive and cohesive environment that promotes individual growth and mutual respect.

Roles Within the Family

Within every family, individuals often assume various roles that contribute to the overall functioning and dynamics of the family unit. These roles may be influenced by factors such as age, gender, personality, and family structure, and they play a crucial role in shaping the way family members interact and relate to one another. In families affected by PDA Autism, the presence of a member with PDA Autism can profoundly impact the distribution of roles and responsibilities, leading to shifts in power dynamics and communication patterns.

One common role within families affected by PDA Autism is that of the primary caregiver, typically assumed by one or both parents. The primary caregiver is responsible for meeting the daily needs of the individual with PDA Autism, including managing demands, providing emotional support, and coordinating services and interventions. This role can be emotionally and physically demanding, requiring patience, resilience, and adaptability in the face of constant challenges and uncertainties.

Another role commonly assumed within families affected by PDA Autism is that of the advocate, tasked with navigating the complex web of services, supports, and educational resources available to individuals with PDA Autism. The advocate serves as a liaison between the family and external systems, advocating for the needs and rights of the individual with PDA Autism and ensuring that they have access to appropriate services and accommodations. This role requires knowledge, persistence, and effective communication skills to navigate bureaucratic systems and overcome barriers to access and inclusion.

In addition to these primary roles, family members may also adopt secondary roles that contribute to the overall functioning of the family unit. Siblings, for example, may assume the role of caregiver, mentor, or protector, depending on their age, personality, and relationship with the individual with PDA Autism. Grandparents, extended family members, and close friends may also play supportive roles within the family system, offering emotional, practical, and financial assistance to ease the burden on primary caregivers.

However, while roles within the family can provide structure and support, they can also become rigid and limiting, leading to feelings of resentment, imbalance, and burnout. It is essential for families affected by PDA Autism to recognize the fluid and evolving nature of roles within the family system and to foster open communication, flexibility, and mutual support to ensure the well-being of all members.

Communication Challenges

Effective communication is essential for maintaining healthy and functional relationships within families. However, in families affected by PDA Autism, communication challenges may arise due to the unique communication style and preferences of individuals with PDA Autism, as well as the impact of demand avoidance and emotional dysregulation on communication dynamics.

One of the primary communication challenges faced by families affected by PDA Autism is the difficulty in deciphering and responding to the communication cues and signals of individuals with

PDA Autism. Individuals with PDA Autism may exhibit atypical patterns of communication, such as echolalia, scripting, or idiosyncratic language, which can be perplexing and challenging for family members to interpret. Furthermore, the demand avoidance characteristic of PDA Autism may manifest in communication avoidance or resistance, leading to breakdowns in communication and frustration for all parties involved.

Moreover, individuals with PDA Autism may struggle with social pragmatics, such as turn-taking, perspective-taking, and understanding nonverbal cues, which can further complicate communication within the family. This difficulty in navigating the nuances of social communication can lead to misunderstandings, misinterpretations, and conflicts, as family members struggle to connect and relate to one another effectively.

Another communication challenge faced by families affected by PDA Autism is the emotional intensity and dysregulation that often accompanies demand avoidance and sensory sensitivities. Individuals with PDA Autism may experience heightened levels of anxiety, frustration, or overwhelm in response to perceived demands or triggers, leading to meltdowns, shutdowns, or withdrawal behaviors.

These emotional outbursts can disrupt communication flow within the family, making it difficult for family members to engage in meaningful dialogue and problem-solving.

To address these communication challenges, families can adopt a variety of strategies and approaches aimed at promoting understanding, empathy, and effective communication. These may include the use of visual supports and aids, such as visual schedules, social stories, and communication boards, to enhance clarity and comprehension. Additionally, practicing active listening, validation, and empathy can foster trust and rapport within the family, creating a supportive and inclusive communication environment where all voices are heard and valued.

Furthermore, it is essential for families to recognize and accommodate the unique communication preferences and needs of individuals with PDA Autism, while also setting clear expectations and boundaries around communication norms and etiquette. By fostering open communication, patience, and flexibility, families can overcome communication challenges and cultivate strong and resilient relationships built on mutual understanding and respect.

Coping Mechanisms

Living with PDA Autism presents unique challenges and stressors for individuals and families alike. Coping mechanisms, or strategies used to manage and mitigate stress and adversity, play a crucial role in promoting resilience and well-being within the family unit. By understanding and implementing effective coping mechanisms, families can navigate the ups and downs of life with PDA Autism with greater ease and adaptability.

One coping mechanism commonly employed by families affected by PDA Autism is the practice of establishing routines and structure within daily life. Establishing predictability and consistency can provide individuals with PDA Autism a sense of stability and control, reducing anxiety and demand avoidance. Families may create visual schedules, use timers or alarms, and implement clear routines for daily activities such as meals, bedtime, and transitions between tasks. By incorporating these strategies into their daily lives, families can minimize the uncertainty and chaos that often accompany the challenges of PDA Autism.

Another essential coping mechanism for families affected by PDA Autism is the practice of self-care.

Caring for a loved one with PDA Autism can be emotionally and physically taxing, requiring significant time, energy, and resources. It is crucial for caregivers to prioritize their own well-being and engage in activities that promote relaxation, stress relief, and personal fulfillment. This may include activities such as exercise, meditation, hobbies, or spending time with friends and loved ones. By investing in their own self-care, caregivers can replenish their reserves and better meet the needs of their family members with PDA Autism.

Additionally, seeking support from others can be a valuable coping mechanism for families affected by PDA Autism. Connecting with other families who share similar experiences can provide validation, empathy, and practical advice for navigating the challenges of PDA Autism. Support groups, online forums, and community organizations dedicated to PDA Autism can offer a sense of belonging and camaraderie, as well as access to valuable resources and information. Moreover, reaching out to friends, family members, or mental health professionals for emotional support and guidance can help families cope with the stress and uncertainty of life with PDA Autism.

Furthermore, practicing mindfulness and acceptance can be powerful coping mechanisms for families affected by PDA Autism. Mindfulness involves cultivating awareness of the present moment, accepting one's thoughts and emotions without judgment, and approaching challenges with compassion and equanimity. By incorporating mindfulness practices into their daily routines, families can reduce stress, enhance resilience, and cultivate a sense of calm amidst the chaos of demand avoidance and emotional dysregulation.

Finally, it is essential for families affected by PDA Autism to remain flexible and adaptable in their approach to coping. The needs and challenges associated with PDA Autism can vary greatly from day to day, requiring families to continually reassess and adjust their coping strategies accordingly. By remaining open to new ideas, experimenting with different approaches, and seeking feedback from each other, families can develop a robust toolkit of coping mechanisms that effectively support their well-being and resilience in the face of PDA Autism.

Chapter 3

Navigating Daily Life

Living with PDA Autism presents unique challenges in navigating daily life, as individuals affected by this condition often struggle with managing demands, sensory sensitivities, and emotional regulation.

Routines and Flexibility

Establishing routines is essential for individuals with PDA Autism, as it provides predictability and structure in their daily lives. Routines help reduce anxiety and uncertainty by outlining expectations and providing a sense of order. However, it is crucial to strike a balance between routines and flexibility, as individuals with PDA Autism may struggle with rigid adherence to schedules and may become overwhelmed by unexpected changes.

Flexibility is key when navigating daily life with PDA Autism, as unexpected events or deviations from routine can trigger anxiety and demand avoidance. Caregivers should aim to introduce flexibility into routines by incorporating opportunities for choice and autonomy, allowing individuals with PDA

Autism to have a sense of control over their environment. Additionally, preparing individuals for changes in routine ahead of time can help mitigate anxiety and improve their ability to cope with unexpected events.

Visual schedules and calendars are valuable tools for promoting both routine and flexibility in daily life. Visual schedules provide a visual representation of daily activities and transitions, helping individuals with PDA Autism anticipate upcoming events and understand the sequence of tasks. By incorporating visual schedules into daily routines, caregivers can empower individuals with PDA Autism to navigate their day with greater independence and confidence.

It is also essential for caregivers to model flexibility and adaptability in their own behavior. By demonstrating resilience in the face of unexpected events and changes in routine, caregivers can help individuals with PDA Autism learn to cope with uncertainty and develop essential life skills.

Sensory Sensitivities

Sensory sensitivities are common among individuals with PDA Autism, as they may experience heightened sensitivity or aversion to sensory stimuli such as light, sound, touch, taste, and smell. Sensory sensitivities can significantly impact daily life, leading to discomfort, anxiety, and demand avoidance in response to overwhelming sensory experiences.

Understanding and accommodating sensory sensitivities is essential for promoting the well-being and functioning of individuals with PDA Autism. Caregivers should be attentive to the specific sensory preferences and aversions of individuals with PDA Autism and work to create environments that support their sensory needs.

One strategy for accommodating sensory sensitivities is the use of sensory-friendly environments. This may involve minimizing sensory triggers such as loud noises, bright lights, or strong smells, and providing opportunities for individuals with PDA Autism to regulate their sensory input. Creating quiet spaces, using soft lighting, and providing sensory tools such as weighted blankets or fidget toys can help individuals with PDA Autism feel more comfortable and relaxed in their environment.

In addition to environmental accommodations, caregivers can also support individuals with PDA Autism in developing sensory regulation strategies. This may include teaching relaxation techniques such as deep breathing or progressive muscle relaxation, as well as encouraging activities that promote sensory integration and modulation, such as swinging, jumping, or brushing.

It is essential for caregivers to approach sensory sensitivities with empathy and understanding, recognizing that each individual may have unique sensory preferences and aversions. By creating a supportive and inclusive environment that honors the sensory needs of individuals with PDA Autism, caregivers can help promote their well-being and participation in daily activities.

Emotional Regulation

Emotional regulation is a significant challenge for individuals with PDA Autism, as they may struggle to understand, express, and manage their emotions effectively. Emotional dysregulation can manifest in a variety of ways, including meltdowns, tantrums, aggression, or withdrawal, and can significantly impact daily functioning and quality of life.

Supporting emotional regulation in individuals with PDA Autism requires a multifaceted approach that addresses the underlying factors contributing to emotional dysregulation. One key strategy is to help individuals identify and label their emotions, providing them with the vocabulary and tools to express their feelings in a constructive manner. Caregivers can use visual supports such as emotion charts or social stories to help individuals with PDA Autism recognize and understand their emotions and learn appropriate ways to express them.

Additionally, caregivers can help individuals with PDA Autism develop coping skills and strategies for managing strong emotions. This may involve teaching relaxation techniques such as deep breathing or mindfulness meditation, as well as providing opportunities for sensory regulation and self-soothing activities. By empowering individuals with PDA Autism to regulate their emotions independently, caregivers can help them build resilience and coping skills that support their overall well-being.

It is also essential for caregivers to create a supportive and validating environment that acknowledges and accepts the emotions of individuals with PDA Autism. By offering empathy, validation, and nonjudgmental support, caregivers can help individuals feel understood and accepted, reducing the likelihood of emotional dysregulation and promoting positive emotional experiences.

Furthermore, caregivers can model healthy emotional regulation skills in their own behavior, demonstrating effective coping strategies and problem-solving techniques in response to challenging situations. By serving as positive role models, caregivers can help individuals with PDA Autism learn to manage their emotions more effectively and navigate daily life with greater confidence and resilience.

School and Education

Navigating the educational system can be particularly challenging for individuals with PDA Autism, as they may encounter difficulties with social communication, demand avoidance, and sensory sensitivities in the school environment. It is essential for caregivers to work collaboratively with educators and school personnel to ensure that the unique needs of individuals with PDA Autism are met and supported.

One key consideration in supporting individuals with PDA Autism in the school setting is the development of individualized education plans (IEPs) or accommodations that address their specific strengths and challenges. This may include modifications to the curriculum, such as providing alternative assignments or reducing the number of demands placed on the individual, as well as accommodations for sensory sensitivities, such as preferential seating or access to sensory breaks.

In addition to academic accommodations, it is crucial for schools to provide support for social and emotional development in individuals with PDA Autism. This may involve the implementation of social skills training programs, peer buddy systems, or counseling services to help individuals with PDA Autism navigate social interactions and develop positive relationships with peers.

Collaboration between caregivers, educators, and school personnel is essential for ensuring the successful implementation of supports and accommodations for individuals with PDA Autism in the school setting. Regular communication and feedback between all stakeholders can help identify emerging challenges, monitor progress, and adjust interventions as needed to meet the evolving needs of the individual.

Furthermore, it is essential for schools to create a supportive and inclusive environment that fosters acceptance and understanding of individuals with PDA Autism. This may involve raising awareness and providing training for school staff on the unique characteristics and needs of individuals with PDA Autism, as well as promoting a culture of empathy, respect, and inclusion among students.

By working collaboratively and proactively to address the academic, social, and emotional needs of individuals with PDA Autism, schools can create an environment where these individuals can thrive and reach their full potential. Through effective collaboration, advocacy, and support, caregivers can help ensure that individuals with PDA Autism receive the education and opportunities they need to succeed in school and beyond.

Chapter 4

Supporting Your Child

Supporting a child with PDA Autism requires a multifaceted approach that addresses their unique strengths, challenges, and needs.

Parenting Strategies

Parenting a child with PDA Autism requires patience, flexibility, and understanding. Effective parenting strategies for children with PDA Autism often focus on establishing clear expectations, promoting positive reinforcement, and fostering a supportive and nurturing environment.

One key parenting strategy for supporting children with PDA Autism is the use of positive reinforcement and praise. Positive reinforcement involves acknowledging and rewarding desirable behaviors, such as following instructions, completing tasks, or engaging in social interactions. By providing positive feedback and reinforcement for desired behaviors, caregivers can help motivate and encourage children with PDA Autism to engage in adaptive and pro-social behaviors.

Additionally, it is essential for caregivers to establish clear and consistent expectations for behavior. Children with PDA Autism may struggle with understanding and complying with rules and expectations, leading to conflicts and misunderstandings. Caregivers can help clarify expectations by using visual supports, such as visual schedules or social stories, to outline rules and routines in a clear and concrete manner. By providing structure and predictability, caregivers can help children with PDA Autism navigate their environment more effectively and reduce anxiety and demand avoidance.

Furthermore, caregivers can support their child's development by fostering opportunities for choice and autonomy. Children with PDA Autism may feel overwhelmed by perceived demands or restrictions on their autonomy, leading to resistance or avoidance behaviors. By offering choices and opportunities for decision-making, caregivers can empower children with PDA Autism to assert control over their environment and feel a sense of ownership and agency.

It is also essential for caregivers to practice patience and flexibility in their approach to parenting children with PDA Autism. Children with PDA Autism may require additional time and support to process information, regulate their emotions, and navigate social interactions. Caregivers can support their child's development by being patient, understanding, and responsive to their needs, adapting their parenting strategies as needed to meet the evolving needs of their child.

Building Self-Esteem

Building self-esteem is essential for children with PDA Autism, as it provides a foundation for positive self-concept, resilience, and well-being. Children with PDA Autism may face unique challenges and barriers to developing self-esteem, including difficulties with social interaction, sensory sensitivities, and demand avoidance. Caregivers can play a critical role in supporting their child's self-esteem by providing encouragement, validation, and opportunities for success.

One key strategy for building self-esteem in children with PDA Autism is to focus on their strengths and interests. Every child has unique talents, abilities, and interests, and caregivers can help their child with PDA Autism discover and nurture these strengths. By providing opportunities for their child to explore and engage in activities that they enjoy and excel in, caregivers can help boost their child's confidence and self-esteem.

Additionally, it is essential for caregivers to provide positive feedback and encouragement for their child's efforts and accomplishments. Children with PDA Autism may struggle with self-doubt and negative self-talk, and caregivers can help counteract these tendencies by offering praise and validation for their child's achievements, no matter how small. By highlighting their child's strengths and successes, caregivers can help build a foundation of self-confidence and resilience that will serve their child well throughout their life.

Furthermore, caregivers can support their child's self-esteem by promoting self-advocacy and autonomy. Children with PDA Autism may face challenges in advocating for their needs and asserting their preferences, and caregivers can help empower their child by teaching them self-advocacy skills and encouraging them to speak up for themselves. By providing opportunities for their child to make choices and decisions, caregivers can help foster a sense of agency and self-efficacy in their child.

It is also essential for caregivers to create a supportive and accepting environment that celebrates their child's uniqueness and individuality. Children with PDA Autism may face stigma, discrimination, and misunderstanding from others, and caregivers can help mitigate these challenges by fostering a sense of belonging and acceptance within the family and community. By modeling empathy, respect, and inclusivity, caregivers can help create a culture of acceptance that nurtures their child's self-esteem and well-being.

Advocating for Your Child

Advocating for a child with PDA Autism is essential for ensuring that their unique needs are met and that they have access to the supports and services they require to thrive. Advocacy involves speaking up on behalf of your child, raising awareness about PDA Autism, and working collaboratively with professionals and organizations to address the challenges and barriers they face.

One key aspect of advocacy for children with PDA Autism is raising awareness and promoting understanding of the condition within the family, school, and community. Many people may be unfamiliar with PDA Autism and its unique characteristics, and caregivers can help educate others by sharing information, resources, and personal experiences. By raising awareness about PDA Autism, caregivers can help promote understanding and acceptance, reduce stigma and discrimination, and create a more supportive and inclusive environment for their child.

Additionally, caregivers can advocate for their child's needs within the educational system by working collaboratively with school personnel to develop individualized education plans (IEPs) or accommodations that address their unique strengths and challenges. This may involve advocating for modifications to the curriculum, providing support for social and emotional development, or ensuring access to appropriate therapies and interventions. By actively participating in the IEP process and advocating for their child's needs, caregivers can help ensure that their child receives the educational support and resources they require to succeed.

Furthermore, caregivers can advocate for their child's needs within the healthcare system by seeking out knowledgeable and supportive professionals who can provide accurate diagnosis, assessment, and treatment of PDA Autism. This may involve seeking referrals to specialists such as developmental pediatricians, psychologists, or occupational therapists who have expertise in PDA Autism and can offer targeted interventions and supports. By advocating for their child's healthcare needs, caregivers can help ensure that their child receives comprehensive and effective care that addresses the full range of their needs.

It is also essential for caregivers to advocate for their child's social and recreational needs by seeking out inclusive activities, programs, and opportunities for their child to participate in. Children with PDA Autism may face barriers to participation in social and recreational activities due to sensory sensitivities, social communication difficulties, or demand avoidance, and caregivers can help break down these barriers by seeking out supportive and accommodating environments where their child can thrive.

Accessing Resources and Support Services

Accessing resources and support services is essential for families of children with PDA Autism to meet their child's unique needs and navigate the challenges associated with the condition. From educational supports to therapeutic interventions, there are various resources and services available to assist families in supporting their child with PDA Autism.

One of the first steps in accessing resources and support services for a child with PDA Autism is obtaining a comprehensive assessment and diagnosis. A thorough assessment by qualified professionals, such as developmental pediatricians, psychologists, or neurologists, can help identify the specific strengths, challenges, and needs of the child, guiding the development of an individualized support plan.

Once a diagnosis has been obtained, families can begin exploring available resources and support services tailored to their child's needs. This may include educational supports such as individualized education plans (IEPs), accommodations, and specialized educational programs designed to meet the unique learning styles and needs of children with PDA Autism. Additionally, families may access therapeutic interventions such as occupational therapy, speech therapy, or behavioral therapy to address sensory sensitivities, communication difficulties, and behavioral challenges associated with PDA Autism.

In addition to educational and therapeutic supports, families may also benefit from accessing support services and programs designed to provide practical assistance and emotional support. This may include parent support groups, online forums, or community organizations dedicated to PDA Autism, where families can connect with others who share similar experiences, share information and resources, and offer mutual support and encouragement.

Furthermore, families may explore financial assistance programs and resources to help alleviate the financial burden associated with raising a child with PDA Autism. This may include accessing government-funded programs such as Medicaid, Supplemental Security Income (SSI), or special education funding, as well as seeking out grants, scholarships, or charitable organizations that provide financial assistance to families of children with special needs.

It is essential for families to conduct thorough research and outreach to identify and access available resources and support services for their child with PDA Autism. This may involve reaching out to healthcare professionals, educators, and other families for recommendations and referrals, as well as conducting online research and exploring community resources and organizations.

Additionally, families may benefit from developing a comprehensive support network of professionals, advocates, and allies who can provide guidance, support, and expertise in navigating the challenges associated with PDA Autism. This may include building relationships with healthcare professionals, educators, therapists, and community organizations that specialize in PDA Autism, as well as connecting with other families who have experience and expertise in supporting children with PDA Autism.

Chapter 5

Sibling Relationships

Sibling relationships play a vital role in the family dynamics of households where a child has PDA Autism. Understanding and supporting these relationships are essential for promoting harmony, empathy, and resilience within the family unit.

Understanding Sibling Dynamics

Sibling dynamics in families affected by PDA Autism are influenced by various factors, including age differences, personality traits, and the unique needs and challenges of the child with PDA Autism. Siblings may experience a range of emotions and responses to having a brother or sister with PDA Autism, including love, admiration, frustration, resentment, and guilt.

Younger siblings may struggle to understand and cope with the demands and idiosyncrasies of their sibling with PDA Autism, while older siblings may feel pressure to assume caregiving responsibilities or act as advocates for their sibling. Siblings may also experience feelings of jealousy or resentment towards their sibling with PDA Autism, particularly if they perceive that their needs or desires are overlooked in favor of their sibling's.

Furthermore, siblings may grapple with feelings of embarrassment or stigma associated with their sibling's behavior or diagnosis, particularly in social or public settings. They may worry about how others perceive their family or fear being judged or excluded because of their sibling's differences.

Understanding these complex sibling dynamics is essential for caregivers and parents to provide appropriate support and guidance to their children. By acknowledging and validating the range of emotions and experiences that siblings may have, parents can create a supportive and open environment where siblings feel safe to express their feelings and concerns.

Supporting Siblings

Supporting siblings of children with PDA Autism involves providing emotional validation, practical support, and opportunities for individual expression and growth. It is essential for parents and caregivers to prioritize the well-being of all their children and create a family culture that values empathy, understanding, and inclusion.

One key strategy for supporting siblings is to provide opportunities for open and honest communication about PDA Autism and its impact on the family. Siblings may have questions or concerns about their sibling's diagnosis, behavior, or needs, and it is essential for parents to provide age-appropriate information and reassurance. By fostering open communication, parents can help siblings develop a better understanding of their sibling's condition and feel more empowered to ask questions and seek support when needed.

Additionally, parents can support siblings by providing opportunities for individual attention, validation, and validation. Siblings may feel overlooked or overshadowed by their sibling with PDA Autism, particularly if their sibling requires a significant amount of time and attention from caregivers. By carving out dedicated time for each child, parents can help siblings feel valued, seen, and appreciated for their unique qualities and contributions.

Furthermore, parents can encourage siblings to pursue their interests, hobbies, and friendships outside of their sibling with PDA Autism. Siblings may benefit from engaging in activities and pursuits that are separate from their sibling with PDA Autism, allowing them to develop their identities, interests, and social connections outside of their family dynamic.

It is also essential for parents to model positive sibling relationships and conflict resolution skills in their own behavior. Siblings learn by example, and parents can set a positive tone for sibling interactions by demonstrating empathy, cooperation, and respect in their interactions with each other and their children. By modeling healthy communication and problem-solving skills, parents can help siblings develop the tools and strategies they need to navigate conflicts and build strong, supportive relationships with each other.

Building Strong Bonds

Building strong bonds between siblings requires intentional effort, empathy, and understanding from parents and caregivers. Despite the challenges posed by PDA Autism, it is possible for siblings to develop deep and meaningful connections with each other, characterized by love, support, and mutual respect.

One key strategy for building strong bonds between siblings is to create opportunities for shared experiences and activities. Siblings may bond over shared interests, hobbies, or experiences, such as playing games, engaging in creative projects, or exploring nature together. By fostering opportunities for siblings to spend quality time together, parents can help strengthen their bond and create lasting memories that they can cherish for years to come.

Additionally, parents can encourage siblings to collaborate and support each other in their interactions with their sibling with PDA Autism. Siblings may benefit from working together to develop strategies for communicating with their sibling, managing challenging behaviors, or supporting their sibling's participation in family activities. By fostering a sense of teamwork and cooperation, parents can help siblings feel empowered and capable of making a positive difference in their sibling's life.

Furthermore, parents can cultivate empathy and understanding between siblings by encouraging them to see the world from each other's perspectives. Siblings may benefit from engaging in activities that promote empathy and perspective-taking, such as role-playing, storytelling, or discussing their sibling's experiences and feelings. By fostering empathy and understanding, parents can help siblings develop a deeper appreciation for each other's unique strengths and challenges and build a foundation of empathy and compassion that will support their relationship throughout their lives.

It is also essential for parents to celebrate and affirm the unique qualities and contributions of each of their children. Siblings may benefit from receiving individual attention, recognition, and praise for their accomplishments and efforts, helping them feel valued and appreciated within the family dynamic. By affirming each child's unique talents, interests, and strengths, parents can help foster a sense of self-worth and belonging that strengthens sibling bonds and promotes positive relationships within the family.

Addressing Sibling Challenges

Despite the potential for strong sibling bonds, siblings of children with PDA Autism may encounter various challenges and stressors that require support and intervention from parents and caregivers. It is essential for parents to be proactive in addressing these challenges and providing their children with the support and resources they need to navigate their sibling relationship successfully.

One common challenge faced by siblings is feelings of jealousy or resentment towards their sibling with PDA Autism. Siblings may feel overlooked or neglected by parents, particularly if their sibling with PDA Autism requires a significant amount of time and attention. Parents can help address these feelings by providing individual attention and validation to each of their children, acknowledging their unique needs and contributions within the family dynamic.

Additionally, siblings may experience feelings of embarrassment or stigma associated with their sibling's behavior or diagnosis, particularly in social or public settings. Parents can help address these feelings by promoting a culture of acceptance, understanding, and inclusivity within the family and community. By fostering open communication and providing opportunities for siblings to share their feelings and concerns, parents can help reduce feelings of shame or isolation and promote a sense of belonging and acceptance for all their children.

Furthermore, siblings may grapple with feelings of guilt or responsibility for their sibling with PDA Autism, particularly if they perceive themselves as failing to protect or support their sibling adequately. Parents can help address these feelings by reassuring their children that they are not responsible for their sibling's condition or behavior and by providing opportunities for siblings to express their feelings and concerns in a safe and supportive environment. By fostering open communication and empathy, parents can help alleviate feelings of guilt or responsibility and promote a sense of mutual support and understanding between siblings.

Chapter 6

Partner Support

Supporting a partner through the challenges of having a child with PDA Autism requires understanding, patience, and effective communication.

Maintaining Connection

Maintaining a strong connection with your partner is essential for navigating the challenges of raising a child with PDA Autism. The stress and demands associated with caring for a child with special needs can take a toll on the relationship, making it crucial for partners to prioritize their connection and communication.

One key strategy for maintaining connection is to carve out dedicated time for quality couple's time. Amidst the demands of caregiving, work, and household responsibilities, it can be easy for partners to neglect their relationship. However, prioritizing regular date nights, shared activities, or simply spending quality time together can help partners stay connected and nurture their bond.

Additionally, effective communication is essential for maintaining connection and resolving conflicts in a constructive manner. Partners should make an effort to listen actively, express their needs and feelings openly, and validate each other's experiences. By creating a safe and supportive space for open communication, partners can strengthen their connection and navigate the challenges of parenting a child with PDA Autism more effectively.

Furthermore, partners can support each other emotionally by offering empathy, validation, and encouragement. Parenting a child with PDA Autism can be emotionally draining, and partners may experience a range of emotions, including stress, frustration, guilt, and sadness. By acknowledging and validating each other's feelings, partners can provide much-needed support and reassurance, fostering resilience and solidarity in their relationship.

It is also essential for partners to prioritize self-care and individual well-being, as maintaining their own physical, emotional, and mental health is essential for supporting each other and their child with PDA Autism effectively. By prioritizing self-care activities such as exercise, relaxation, hobbies, and social connections, partners can replenish their reserves and better cope with the demands of caregiving.

Coping Strategies for Couples

Coping with the stress and challenges of parenting a child with PDA Autism requires effective coping strategies and resilience-building techniques. Partners can support each other by developing coping strategies that promote emotional well-being, reduce stress, and enhance resilience in the face of adversity.

One key coping strategy for couples is to practice mindfulness and stress reduction techniques. Mindfulness involves cultivating awareness of the present moment, accepting one's thoughts and emotions without judgment, and approaching challenges with equanimity and compassion. Partners can practice mindfulness together through activities such as meditation, deep breathing exercises, or mindfulness walks, helping them reduce stress and foster a sense of calm amidst the chaos of caregiving.

Additionally, couples can benefit from developing a support network of family, friends, and professionals who can provide practical assistance, emotional support, and guidance. Sharing their experiences and challenges with trusted individuals can help partners feel less isolated and overwhelmed, providing a valuable source of encouragement and validation.

Furthermore, couples can benefit from setting realistic expectations and boundaries around their caregiving responsibilities. Parenting a child with PDA Autism can be demanding and unpredictable, and partners may need to adjust their expectations and priorities accordingly. By setting realistic goals, delegating tasks, and seeking help when needed, partners can reduce stress and prevent burnout in their caregiving role.

It is also essential for couples to prioritize their relationship and make time for regular check-ins and discussions about their experiences, feelings, and needs. Partners can benefit from setting aside dedicated time for communication, problem-solving, and emotional connection, helping them stay connected and aligned in their caregiving approach.

Balancing Responsibilities

Balancing responsibilities between partners is essential for maintaining harmony and efficiency in caregiving for a child with PDA Autism. Partners must work together to divide tasks, share responsibilities, and support each other in meeting the needs of their child and family.

One key strategy for balancing responsibilities is to identify each partner's strengths, preferences, and areas of expertise. Partners may have different strengths and skills that they can leverage in their caregiving role, such as one partner being more adept at managing appointments and paperwork, while the other excels at providing emotional support and sensory regulation.

Additionally, partners can benefit from dividing tasks and responsibilities based on their availability, energy levels, and other commitments. By collaborating to create a balanced schedule that takes into account each partner's needs and preferences, partners can ensure that caregiving responsibilities are shared fairly and efficiently.

Furthermore, partners can support each other by offering flexibility and understanding when unexpected challenges arise. Parenting a child with PDA Autism can be unpredictable, and partners may need to adjust their schedules and priorities accordingly. By communicating openly and being willing to adapt to changing circumstances, partners can navigate the demands of caregiving with greater ease and flexibility.

It is also essential for partners to communicate openly and regularly about their needs, boundaries, and expectations regarding caregiving responsibilities. By having honest discussions about their roles and responsibilities, partners can ensure that they are on the same page and address any potential conflicts or misunderstandings proactively.

Seeking External Support

Seeking external support is essential for partners in families affected by PDA Autism to access the resources, guidance, and assistance they need to navigate the challenges of caregiving effectively. Partners can benefit from reaching out to professionals, support groups, and community organizations that specialize in PDA Autism and can provide valuable support and resources.

One key source of external support for partners is professional guidance from therapists, counselors, or psychologists who specialize in working with families affected by PDA Autism. These professionals can provide individual or couples therapy to help partners process their emotions, develop coping strategies, and strengthen their relationship. Additionally, they can offer guidance and support in navigating the challenges of parenting a child with PDA Autism and accessing appropriate resources and interventions.

Furthermore, partners can benefit from connecting with support groups or online forums for families affected by PDA Autism. These groups provide a valuable source of peer support, empathy, and understanding, as well as access to information, resources, and practical advice. By sharing their experiences and challenges with other families who understand their journey, partners can feel less isolated and overwhelmed, finding solace and validation in knowing that they are not alone in their experiences.

Moreover, seeking support from family and friends can also be beneficial for partners in families affected by PDA Autism. Loved ones can provide practical assistance with caregiving tasks, offer emotional support and encouragement, and provide respite care to give partners a much-needed break. By reaching out to their support network, partners can lighten their caregiving load and find comfort in knowing that they have people they can rely on during challenging times.

Additionally, partners can benefit from accessing community organizations and resources that specialize in providing support and services to families affected by PDA Autism. These organizations may offer educational workshops, support groups, recreational programs, and advocacy services tailored to the needs of families raising children with PDA Autism. By connecting with these organizations, partners can access valuable resources, information, and support that can help them navigate the challenges of caregiving more effectively.

Chapter 7

Extended Family and Community

In the journey of raising a child with PDA Autism, the support and understanding of extended family members and the wider community play a vital role.

Educating Extended Family Members

Many extended family members may be unfamiliar with PDA Autism and its unique characteristics, leading to misunderstandings, misconceptions, and stigma. Parents can play a proactive role in educating their extended family members by providing information, resources, and personal insights into their child's diagnosis and needs.

One effective strategy for educating extended family members is to initiate open and honest conversations about PDA Autism. Parents can share information about their child's diagnosis, characteristics, and challenges, as well as their family's experiences and journey. By providing firsthand insights and personal anecdotes, parents can help demystify PDA Autism and dispel misconceptions, fostering greater understanding and empathy among extended family members.

Additionally, parents can provide educational materials and resources to extended family members to help them learn more about PDA Autism. This may include sharing articles, books, websites, or videos that provide information about PDA Autism, its characteristics, and effective strategies for supporting individuals with the condition. By equipping extended family members with accurate and reliable information, parents can empower them to better understand and support their child with PDA Autism.

Furthermore, parents can encourage extended family members to ask questions and seek clarification about PDA Autism. Open dialogue and communication are essential for promoting understanding and addressing any misconceptions or concerns that extended family members may have. By creating a safe and supportive space for discussion, parents can foster meaningful conversations that promote empathy, awareness, and support within the extended family.

It is also essential for parents to advocate for their child's needs and preferences within the extended family, ensuring that family gatherings, events, and activities are inclusive and accommodating of their child with PDA Autism. This may involve discussing potential accommodations or modifications to family gatherings to support their child's sensory sensitivities, communication preferences, or social comfort levels. By advocating for their child's needs within the extended family, parents can help create a supportive and inclusive environment that celebrates their child's uniqueness and fosters acceptance and understanding of PDA Autism.

In summary, educating extended family members about PDA Autism involves initiating open and honest conversations, providing educational materials and resources, encouraging questions and dialogue, and advocating for inclusivity and accommodation within the extended family. By equipping extended family members with accurate information and fostering understanding and empathy, parents can cultivate a supportive and inclusive family environment that promotes the well-being and acceptance of their child with PDA Autism.

Creating Supportive Networks

Creating supportive networks within the extended family and community is essential for providing families affected by PDA Autism with the support, understanding, and resources they need to navigate the challenges of raising a child with the condition. Supportive networks can provide emotional validation, practical assistance, and opportunities for connection and shared experiences, helping families feel less isolated and overwhelmed.

One effective strategy for creating supportive networks is to reach out to other families affected by PDA Autism within the extended family or community. Connecting with other families who understand the challenges and experiences of raising a child with PDA Autism can provide valuable peer support, empathy, and validation. Parents can share information, resources, and strategies for coping with the demands of caregiving, as well as offer encouragement and solidarity during challenging times.

Additionally, parents can benefit from joining support groups or online forums for families affected by PDA Autism. These groups provide a valuable source of peer support, information, and advice, as well as opportunities for connection and shared experiences. By participating in support groups, parents can access a supportive community of individuals who understand their journey and can offer guidance, encouragement, and empathy.

Furthermore, parents can create supportive networks within their local community by connecting with professionals, educators, and service providers who specialize in PDA Autism. These individuals can offer valuable support, guidance, and resources to help families navigate the challenges of raising a child with PDA Autism effectively. By building relationships with professionals and service providers, parents can access specialized interventions, therapies, and supports that address their child's unique needs and promote their well-being.

It is also essential for parents to cultivate supportive relationships with friends, neighbors, and members of their community who can offer practical assistance, emotional support, and opportunities for connection and socialization. Whether it's arranging playdates, offering respite care, or providing a listening ear, friends and neighbors can play a crucial role in helping families affected by PDA

Autism feel supported and connected within their community.

In summary, creating supportive networks within the extended family and community involves reaching out to other families affected by PDA Autism, joining support groups or online forums, connecting with professionals and service providers, and cultivating supportive relationships with friends, neighbors, and community members. By building a network of support, understanding, and resources, families can navigate the challenges of raising a child with PDA Autism more effectively and feel less isolated and overwhelmed in their caregiving journey.

Community Resources and Programs

Accessing community resources and programs is essential for families affected by PDA Autism to access the support, services, and opportunities they need to promote their child's well-being and development. Community resources and programs can provide a wide range of supports, including educational interventions, therapeutic services, recreational activities, and advocacy initiatives, tailored to the needs of individuals with PDA Autism and their families.

One key resource for families affected by PDA Autism is early intervention services, which provide specialized support and interventions to promote the development and well-being of young children with developmental delays or disabilities. Early intervention services may include speech therapy, occupational therapy, physical therapy, and developmental assessments, tailored to the unique needs of children with PDA Autism and their families. By accessing early intervention services, families can access the supports and interventions they need to promote their child's development and address any challenges or delays they may be experiencing.

Additionally, families can benefit from accessing educational supports and accommodations through their local school district or educational system. Individuals with PDA Autism may be eligible for special education services, accommodations, or supports to help them access the curriculum, participate in school activities, and reach their academic potential. By collaborating with educators and school personnel, families can develop individualized education plans (IEPs) or accommodations that address their child's unique strengths and challenges, promoting their academic success and well-being.

Furthermore, families can access therapeutic services and interventions through community-based organizations, clinics, or private practitioners. Therapeutic interventions such as behavioral therapy, social skills training, sensory integration therapy, and cognitive-behavioral therapy can help individuals with PDA Autism develop essential skills, cope with challenges, and improve their overall functioning and quality of life. By accessing therapeutic services, families can access the specialized supports and interventions they need to address their child's unique needs and promote their well-being and development.

It is also essential for families to explore recreational programs and activities within their community that are inclusive and accommodating of individuals with PDA Autism. Many community organizations, parks and recreation departments, and nonprofit organizations offer recreational programs, clubs, or activities specifically designed for individuals with special needs, including PDA Autism. By participating in these programs, individuals with PDA Autism can access opportunities for socialization, recreation, and skill-building in a supportive and inclusive environment.

Advocating for Awareness and Understanding

Advocating for awareness and understanding of PDA Autism within the community is essential for promoting acceptance, inclusion, and support for individuals with the condition and their families. Many members of the community may be unfamiliar with PDA Autism and its unique characteristics, leading to misunderstandings, misconceptions, and stigma. Parents and caregivers can play a proactive role in advocating for awareness and understanding by raising awareness, dispelling myths, and promoting acceptance and inclusion within the community.

One effective strategy for advocating for awareness and understanding is to share personal stories and experiences about PDA Autism with others in the community. By sharing their experiences and insights, parents and caregivers can help educate others about the challenges and strengths of individuals with PDA Autism and their families, fostering empathy, understanding, and support within the community.

Additionally, parents and caregivers can advocate for awareness and understanding of PDA Autism by participating in community events, workshops, or presentations that focus on autism awareness and acceptance. By volunteering to speak at community events or organizations, parents and caregivers can raise awareness about PDA Autism, share information and resources, and promote acceptance and inclusion within the community.

Furthermore, parents and caregivers can advocate for awareness and understanding of PDA Autism within educational settings, workplaces, and other community organizations. By collaborating with educators, employers, and community leaders, parents and caregivers can raise awareness about PDA Autism, advocate for accommodations and supports, and promote inclusive practices that support the needs of individuals with the condition and their families.

It is also essential for parents and caregivers to advocate for policy changes and initiatives that promote awareness, acceptance, and inclusion of individuals with PDA Autism within the community. This may include advocating for increased funding for autism research, supporting initiatives that promote inclusive education and employment opportunities, and advocating for policies that protect the rights and dignity of individuals with autism and their families.

Chapter 8

Embracing Humor and Compassion

In the journey of navigating PDA Autism within the family, embracing humor and compassion can be powerful tools for promoting resilience, fostering understanding, and finding joy amidst the challenges.

Finding Joy in Everyday Moments

Even amidst the challenges of PDA Autism, there are countless opportunities to find joy and laughter in everyday moments. For example, imagine a family sitting down for dinner together. The child with PDA Autism, let's call him Alex, has a particular aversion to certain textures and smells of food, making mealtime a stressful experience for everyone. Instead of focusing on the difficulties, the family decides to turn mealtime into a fun and interactive experience. They create a "food adventure" game where each family member takes turns describing a food item in a silly or exaggerated way, and Alex gets to guess what it is. This not only helps distract Alex from his sensory aversions but also turns mealtime into a lighthearted and enjoyable experience for the entire family.

Similarly, finding joy in everyday moments can involve embracing the unique interests and passions of the child with PDA Autism. For instance, imagine a family spending a Saturday afternoon at the park. While other children are playing on the swings or climbing on the jungle gym, Alex is captivated by the complex patterns and textures of the leaves on the trees. Instead of rushing him to join the other children, the family encourages Alex to explore his interests and spend time observing nature. They bring along a sketchbook and colored pencils so Alex can document his observations and create his own artwork inspired by nature. This not only allows Alex to engage in an activity he loves but also fosters a sense of connection and joy within the family as they share in Alex's passion and creativity.

Celebrating Differences

Celebrating the differences of individuals with PDA Autism is essential for fostering acceptance, inclusion, and self-confidence. Rather than focusing on what individuals with PDA Autism cannot do, it's important to recognize and celebrate their unique strengths, talents, and perspectives. For example, imagine a school talent show where students are showcasing their abilities in singing, dancing, and playing musical instruments. While Alex may not feel comfortable performing on stage in front of a large audience, he has a remarkable talent for memorizing and reciting facts about his favorite topic: dinosaurs. Instead of feeling discouraged, Alex's family encourages him to share his passion for dinosaurs with his classmates in a unique and creative way. They help him create a "Dino Quiz" game where he challenges his classmates to answer trivia questions about dinosaurs. This not only allows Alex to showcase his knowledge and passion but also fosters a sense of pride and accomplishment as he shares his interests with others.

Similarly, celebrating differences can involve embracing the unique communication styles and preferences of individuals with PDA Autism. For instance, imagine a family gathering where relatives are engaged in lively conversations and storytelling. While some family members may find it challenging to understand Alex's nonverbal communication cues or repetitive speech patterns, his family members make an effort to listen attentively and respond with patience and understanding. They recognize that Alex communicates in his own unique way and make an effort to accommodate his preferences and needs. Instead of viewing Alex's communication differences as limitations, they celebrate his ability to express himself in his own authentic way, fostering acceptance and inclusivity within the family.

Fostering Resilience

Fostering resilience in individuals with PDA Autism involves providing them with the tools, support, and opportunities they need to navigate challenges, cope with adversity, and bounce back from setbacks. For example, imagine Alex is preparing to attend a birthday party for one of his classmates. While he is excited about the opportunity to socialize and participate in the festivities, he also feels anxious about the unfamiliar environment and social expectations. Instead of avoiding the party altogether, Alex's family helps him develop a resilience plan to cope with his anxiety and navigate the event successfully. They practice social scripts and role-play different scenarios to help Alex feel more confident and prepared. They also create a "comfort kit" containing items that help calm and ground Alex, such as sensory toys, headphones, and a favorite book. With the support and guidance of his family, Alex attends the party and navigates the social interactions with resilience and confidence, building his self-esteem and sense of mastery in the process.

Similarly, fostering resilience can involve helping individuals with PDA Autism develop coping strategies and self-regulation techniques to manage stress and regulate their emotions. For instance, imagine Alex is feeling overwhelmed and agitated after a long day at school. Instead of reacting impulsively or becoming dysregulated, he takes a break in his "calm corner" at home, where he can engage in calming activities such as deep breathing exercises, sensory play, or listening to music. His family members respect his need for space and provide him with support and encouragement as he practices his coping strategies. Over time, Alex learns to recognize his own signs of stress and implement coping strategies independently, fostering a sense of empowerment and resilience in managing his emotions and behaviors.

Moreover, fostering resilience in individuals with PDA Autism involves providing them with opportunities to build confidence and competence in various areas of their lives. For example, imagine

Alex expressing an interest in learning to ride a bike, despite his initial apprehension and fear of falling. His family supports his interest by gradually introducing him to biking in a safe and supportive environment, such as a quiet park with a flat, smooth surface. They provide him with a balance bike to help him develop his balance and coordination at his own pace, celebrating each small achievement along the way. With patience, encouragement, and support from his family, Alex gradually builds his confidence and skills, eventually mastering the art of riding a bike and experiencing a sense of accomplishment and pride in his abilities.

Cultivating a Positive Outlook

Cultivating a positive outlook involves fostering optimism, hope, and gratitude in individuals with PDA Autism and their families, even in the face of challenges and adversity. For example, imagine Alex is facing a particularly challenging day at school, where he experiences sensory overload and struggles to regulate his emotions. Instead of dwelling on the difficulties of the day, his family encourages him to reflect on the positive aspects of his day, such as moments of connection with classmates, accomplishments in his schoolwork, or enjoyable sensory experiences during recess. They create a "gratitude jar" where Alex can write down things he is grateful for each day, no matter how small, and revisit them when he needs a reminder of the positive aspects of his life. By focusing on the positive aspects of his day, Alex learns to reframe challenges as opportunities for growth and resilience, fostering a sense of optimism and hope for the future.

Similarly, cultivating a positive outlook can involve finding humor and levity in challenging situations, even amidst the stress and uncertainty of daily life. For instance, imagine Alex is feeling anxious about an upcoming dentist appointment, where he will need to undergo a dental procedure that he finds uncomfortable and frightening. Instead of allowing anxiety to overshadow the experience, his family helps him approach the appointment with a sense of humor and lightheartedness. They create a "dentist survival kit" containing items that make Alex feel calm and comforted, such as his favorite stuffed animal, headphones to listen to music, and a silly joke book to distract him during the procedure. By infusing humor and levity into the experience, Alex feels more relaxed and at ease, turning what could have been a stressful experience into a positive and even enjoyable one.

Conclusion

The journey of understanding, supporting, and embracing the unique dynamics of PDA Autism within the family is both challenging and rewarding. Through the chapters explored in this handbook, we've delved into the various facets of PDA Autism, from its characteristics and impact on family dynamics to practical strategies for navigating daily life and fostering support networks. Each chapter has provided valuable insights, practical advice, and real-life scenarios to help families navigate the complexities of PDA Autism with compassion, resilience, and humor.

Throughout this handbook, the importance of empathy, understanding, and acceptance has been emphasized as foundational pillars for supporting individuals with PDA Autism and their families. By fostering open communication, creating supportive environments, and celebrating the unique strengths and differences of individuals with PDA Autism, families can cultivate a sense of belonging, resilience, and well-being.

Moreover, the significance of humor and compassion in navigating the challenges of PDA Autism cannot be overstated. By finding joy in everyday moments, celebrating differences, fostering resilience, and cultivating a positive outlook, families can create a nurturing and uplifting environment that promotes acceptance, connection, and growth.

As families continue on their journey of supporting a loved one with PDA Autism, it's essential to remember that each step, no matter how small, contributes to a tapestry of understanding, compassion, and resilience. By embracing the journey with an open heart and a willingness to learn and grow, families can navigate the complexities of PDA Autism with grace, humor, and compassion, fostering a sense of unity, strength, and love within the family unit.

www.ingramcontent.com/pod-product-compliance
Lightning Source LLC
Chambersburg PA
CBHW050236230526
45470CB00005B/1985